SCIATICA HOME EXERCISES & TREATMENT

WHITLEY SMITH

TABLE OF CONTENT

INTRODUCTION

This book is your comprehensive guide to understanding sciatica and its treatments. In this book, you will find simple yet effective exercises and treatments that can be done at home to help ease the pain of sciatica. We will discuss the causes of sciatica, its symptoms, risk factors, and the various treatments and exercises that can help. You will also learn how to prevent and manage sciatica flare-ups, as well as how to identify any underlying conditions that may be contributing to your sciatica. With this book, you will gain the knowledge and confidence to take control of your sciatica and start feeling better.

SCIATICA PAIN

The term "sciatica" refers to pain felt along the sciatic nerve. The lengthiest and broadest nerve in the human body is the sciatic nerve. The sciatic nerve is in charge of regulating some number of lower leg muscles.

Additionally it provides sensation to the skin, the foot, and the bulk of the lower leg. Up to forty percent of people, according to some professionals, will encounter sciatica at least once in their lives. It is worthy to know that sciatica is a symptom and not a disease.

This type of severe nerve problem and irritation can be quite burdensome because the spinal nerve oversees managing the activities of various muscles in the legs and hips. Nevertheless, one must keep in mind that there is no consistency in the intensity and signs of various sciatica incidents. The pain can vary from low aches, joint pain or paralysis, and a prickling along the nerve area to much more extreme pain that feels like acute electrocution. In a few instances, the piercing pain intensifies with the smallest activity, leaving the victim unable to move their feet, bend knees and toes, walk, or move their toes.

It mostly affects people between the ages of thirty and fifty. Sometimes, it only attacks one part of the body, but it can be intense and exhausting.

Symptoms of Sciatica Nerve Pain

Based on the intensity of your situation, the symptoms of sciatic nerve pain can change. You should speak with your doctor if you are suffering serious sciatic nerve pain. Some of the symptoms of sciatica is listed below for your reference:

- ✓ Pain that extends from your lower spine down your leg's back and to your buttocks.

- ✓ Irritation anywhere along the nerve system.

- ✓ Burning Sensation

- ✓ Agonizing pain.

- ✓ Numbness.

- ✓ Tingling effect

- ✓ Weakness of the muscle.

- ✓ Persistent pain in just one side of the leg or buttock.

- ✓ Sharp pain.

✓ Extreme pain in one leg that makes it difficult to stand or walk.

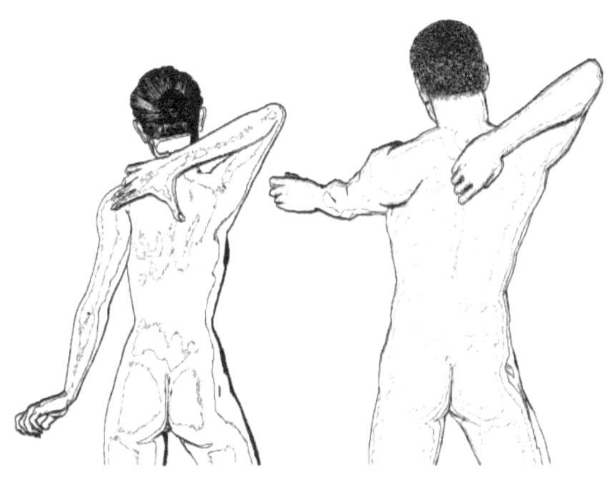

CAUSES OF SCIATICA PAIN

Sciatica pain is a usual symptom of several health conditions. Almost all occurrences of sciatica pain can be tracked down to a slipped disc in the lower back. Your vertebral body is made up of three parts: vertebra, nerves, and skeleton. The disks are made of cardboard, yet they can still cause injury. A disk becomes ruptured when it is forced out of place, placing pressure on the sciatica nerve. You can find some of the causes of Sciatica pain below:

- ✓ The most frequent cause of sciatica is a ruptured disk. These discs have the tendency to rupture as people age, allowing the fluid to leak out.

- ✓ A spinal injury or infection

- ✓ Degenerative disc disease includes the progressive deterioration of the articulating discs between the spinal vertebrae.

- ✓ Growth of bone spurs or bone overgrowths on your vertebrae.

- ✓ Pregnancy

- ✓ Spinal stenosis or narrowing of the spinal canal

- ✓ Isthmic spondylolisthesis, a vertebra slips forward overlapping another one.

- ✓ Piriformis syndrome, when the piriformis muscle, situated deep in the buttocks, spasms is putting pressure on the adjoining sciatic nerve.

- ✓ Pelvic injury or fracture

✓ Tumors

✓ Lumbar spinal stenosis - narrowing of the spinal cord and lower back.

✓ Spondylolisthesis - a disk slips forward over the vertebra below it.

✓ Tumors within the spine may compress the root of the sciatic nerve.

✓ An infection can damage and ultimately affect the spine.

✓ If you have suffered a severe back injury you may experience sciatica pain.

✓ Cauda equine syndrome - serious condition that affects the nerves in the lower part of the spinal cord.

SCIATICA PAIN RISK FACTORS & COMPLICATIONS

Numerous acts can lead to an increased risk of developing sciatica pain.

- ✓ Age is one of the most unavoidable. The most frequent causes of sciatica are changes in the spine brought on by aging, such as slipped discs and bone spurs.

- ✓ Obesity is another factor. The strain on your spine rises when you add a lot of weight. Added stress may add to the spinal changes that activate sciatica pain.

- ✓ Your line of work may also be viewed as a risk factor for sciatica. The pain could result from any task that needs you to strain your back, handle heavy things, or operate a vehicle on the road for an extended period.

Uncontrolled sciatica can have consequences that most individuals could fully recover from.

Nevertheless, if you encounter any of the following, you should seek immediate medical attention:

- ✓ Loss of sensation in the affected leg

- ✓ Weakness in the affected leg

- ✓ Loss of bowel or bladder function.

SCIATICA PAIN TREATMENT

There are many treatment options accessible because sciatica pain is such a prevalent occurrence. You can discuss medical symptoms and treatments with your doctor. These will be quite efficient and help to be correctly diagnosed in order to have the best sciatica relief.

Medication

The categories of pharmaceuticals that could be prescribed for sciatica pain are tricyclic anti-depressants, anti-seizure drugs, anti-inflammatory drugs, and muscle relaxants. These will lessen the discomfort and numbness associated with sciatica.

Physical Therapy

You may be allocated a rehabilitation program when your intense pain has improved. This will aid in averting future injuries. This almost always includes physical pain relief exercises to restore your posture and strengthen the muscles stabilizing your back. It could also increase your flexibility.

Steroid Injections

Your doctor may prescribe you an injection of a corticosteroid medication in a few specific circumstances. This injection would be administered in the vicinity of the concerned nerve roof. By suppressing inflammation around the affected nerve, corticosteroids will help lessen the pain. Normally, the impacts fade off after a few months. Due to the risk of serious side effects from taking steroids, you can't receive too many of these shots. When injections happen too often, the risk of these detrimental effects increases.

This is typically done when the nerve creates serious weakness, a loss of bowel or bladder control, or when the pain does not get better using other treatments. The bone spur or herniated disk that is resting on the strained nerve can be eliminated by surgeons. Due to a lengthy recuperation period, doctors usually try to avoid surgery.

SCIATICA PAIN HOME REMEDIES

Luckily, there is a sciatica pain treatment that may be carried out at home. It's crucial that you see a doctor if any of these at-home solutions don't help your pain decrease. If the pain worsens, you might have a more serious situation than you initially believed. The following are some at-home remedies for treating sciatica.

Discontinue Gym Workouts

Exercise is beneficial, but it should not result in more serious problems. Your spinal nerve will be put under more stress than usual by some exercises. The natural movement patterns of your body will typically be restricted by most gym equipment. Use natural activities like walking, running, and swimming to replace workouts in the gym.

Do Stretching Exercises

A few problems with the sciatica nerves can be addressed by stretching. Small amounts of stretching can ease the stress on the limbs and the heart. This will lead to sciatica relief.

Practice Yoga

Yoga is connected to both stretching and a holistic medical system. It will help increase flexibility and correct incorrect postures that lead to spinal issues. There are several positions that are suggested for physical pain relief activities.

Use a Natural Pain Relieve

Ginger tea and turmeric milk are also excellent anti-inflammatories.

A fantastic sciatica treatment option may be a deep massage. The massage will follow the nerve's natural path and massage the blood flow. The problem will not be completely solved by this temporary fix. You should seek out a knowledgeable masseuse who is familiar with the right procedure.

SCIATICA EXERCISES FOR QUICK PAIN RELIEF

Several exercises canare several exercises that can offer quick and simple relief for sciatica pain. They can be completed at home and within a short amount of time. They are straightforward enough that you don't need to be an expert to execute them. Below are some of these exercises.

Reclining Pigeon Pose

Directions

- ✓ Lying on your back, raise your right leg to a right angle.

- ✓ Grab the two hands at the back of the thigh.

- ✓ Elevate your left leg, then position your right ankle on top of your left knee.

- ✓ Wait for for a while.

- ✓ Then release and redo the process with the other leg.

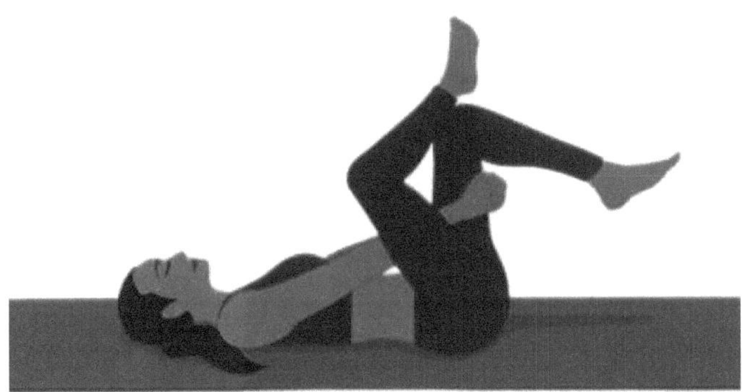

Sitting Pigeon Pose

Directions

- ✓ Stretch your legs out straight and bring your feet together as you sit on the ground.

- ✓ The right ankle is crossed over the left knee when the right leg is bent.

✓ Let the upper body softly descend toward the thigh as you bend forward at the hips.

✓ Based on your ease, maintain the stretch for fifteen seconds.

✓ Do the stretch on the opposite side as you gradually let go of the hold.

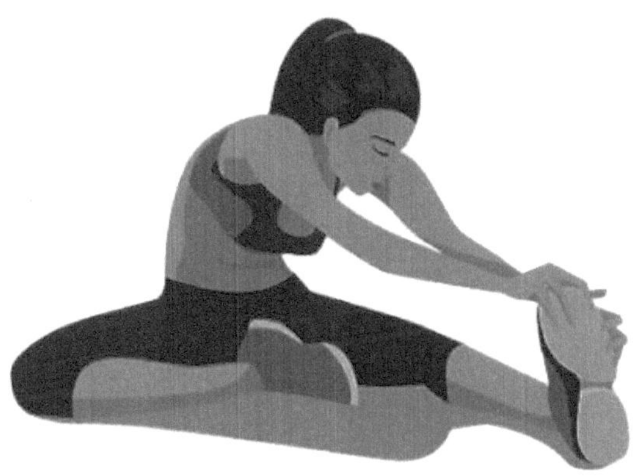

Forward Pigeon Pose

Directions

- ✓ On all fours, kneel on the ground.

- ✓ Take up your right leg and advance it forward on the floor in front of you.

- ✓ Extend your left leg out all the way behind you on the ground, with the tip of your feet on the ground and your toes directed back.

- ✓ Slowly move your body weight from your arms to your legs such that your legs are carrying your weight.

- ✓ Get comfortable by taking a deep breath.

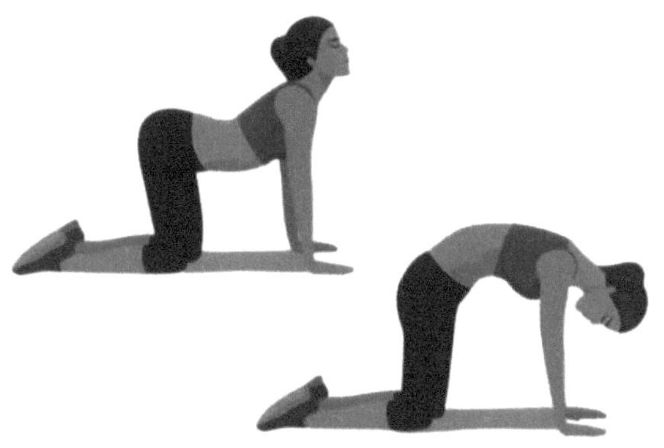

Knee to Chest Pose

Directions

- ✓ Lying on your back with your legs curved in such a way that your knees point to the sky and your feet lay flat on the floor.

- ✓ With the other foot still on the ground, lift one knee to the chest.

✓ Raise the knee to the chest for as long as it
feels safe, up to twenty seconds.

✓ Relax the leg gradually, then do the same
with the opposite leg.

✓ For each leg, strive for Three repetitions.

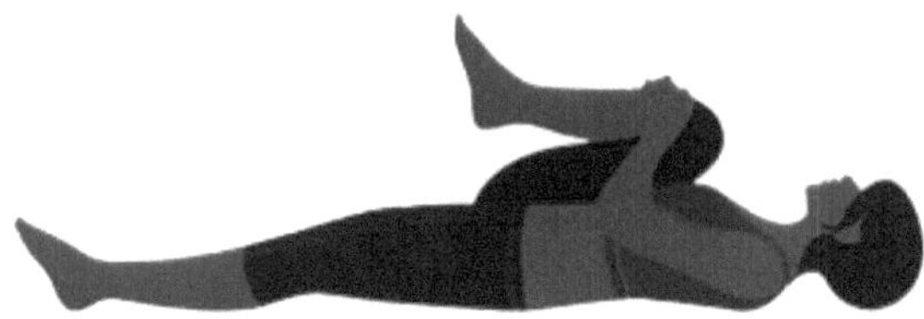

Sitting Spinal Stretch

Directions

✓ Sitting on the floor, legs stretched out and
your feet curved upward.

✓ Flex your right knee and bring your foot flat on the floor.

✓ To assist you in naturally moving your body to the right, bring your left elbow on the outside of your right knee.

✓ Wait for thirty seconds, then repeat three times before changing sides.

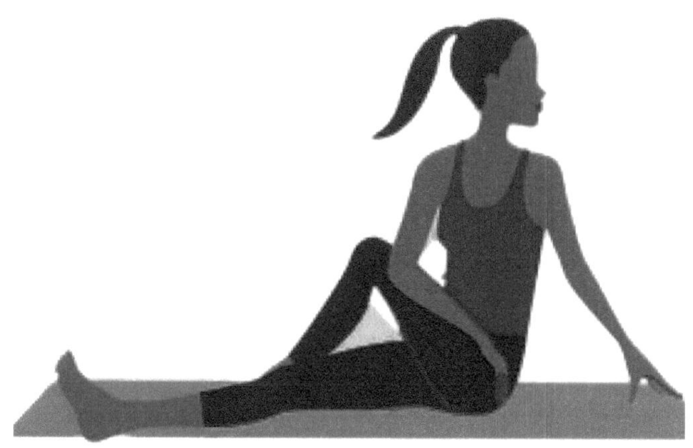

HOW TO RELIEVE SCIATICA NERVE PAIN NATURALLY

Even thoughthe fact that there are numerous traditional remedies for sciatica, they may only temporarily lessen the pain. Unfortunately, most steroid injections can have devastating side effects.

To lessen inflammation and pressure on the irritated sciatic nerve, you might use several home remedies and natural treatments. The problem usually resolves itself with time. The home treatments for sciatica are listed below:

Utilizing hot or cold compresses can help relieve sciatica pain and swelling. The sciatic nerve may be compressed by tense muscles, which are relieved with heat therapy. Cold treatment decreases swelling around the nerve and deaden the pain. Alternating between hot and cold, starting with the hot compressor and finishing with the cold compressor, is another option. For the hot compressor, it is more effective to use steamed towel.

Directions

- ✓ For fifteen minutes, put a steamed towel or cold pack on the targeted area.

✓ Until you notice improvement, repeat this
action every few hours.

✓ Use a warm compressor if you have
circulatory issues.

Low Back Massage

Specifically, if the issue is brought on by a muscular spasm, treatment can ease sciatica pain and help the body to cure itself. According to research, massage therapy helps minimize chronic low back pain. A common sign of sciatica is low back pain.

Directions

✓ Three times each day, until you experience
relief, massage the affected area with an oil
that has anti-inflammatory properties to help
relieve sciatica pain and inflammation.

✓ The addition of three tablespoons of nutmeg powder to one cup of sesame oil is another option.

✓ Warm up the mix. Let it cools completely and massage the damaged area with it. Do this till you feel better.

✓ You may also think about trigger-point (lower back, buttock, and side of the thigh) massage therapy, preferably once daily.

Exercises to Relieve the Pain

✓ Retaining regular activities is incredibly useful for trying to deal with sciatica. After a sciatica episode, victims can start a normal workout regimen to strengthen their abdominal and back muscles. The core muscles can be strengthened to assist in swift recovery.

✓ To help lessen the discomfort of the sciatic nerve and improve the flexibility of your lower back, you can do the Knee to Chest Stretch.

✓ In order to alleviate sciatica and lower back pain, patients can also engage in workouts like spinal rolling, knee squatting, floor twists, back bluffs, back extensions, and certain yoga poses such as the cat-cow and pigeon poses.

Note: To assist you to establish the appropriate workout plan for your circumstances, see medical therapist.

Turmeric has anti-inflammatory properties, making it an efficient organic treatment for sciatica. Turmeric has a substance referred to as curcumin, which aids in lessening nerve pain and swelling.

Directions

- ✓ To one cup of milk, add one teaspoon of turmeric.

- ✓ Add a little cinnamon tick. Heat the solution.

- ✓ Consume this nutritional drink once or twice a day until you feel better.

- ✓ You may want to add honey.

Note: For people taking blood thinners or drugs for diabetes, Turmeric may not be appropriate. Additionally, people dealing with gallstones ought to shun it.

Spinal Manipulation

A growing number of people are turning to chiropractic care as a natural remedy for neck and back pain.

Spinal manipulative therapy is another name for spinal manipulation. It's a procedure where experts administer a controlled shove to a joint of your spine using their hands or a tool. The shove pushes the joint further than it would on by itself, albeit the force applied can differ.

The majority of spinal manipulations are performed by chiropractors, while osteopathic doctors and physical therapists are also qualified to do this type of the procedure.

The manipulation of the spine involves quick, rapid motions. When you think about a chiropractic adjustment, you probably hear that familiar "crack" sound, and many sufferers claim to experience instant, pleasurable ease. The procedure promotes a normal blood flow, helps ease tension in the nearby soft tissue, and induces calmness.

It is intended to ease joint pressure, lessen inflammation, and enhance nerve function. Pain in the back, neck, shoulder, and head is frequently treated with it.

Consult a specialist in chiropractic medicine for the best course of treatment for your sciatica pain, based on the precise cause.

Acupuncture

Another efficient natural remedy to alleviate sciatica pain, calm the muscles, and assist in self-healing is acupuncture. A theory states that stimulating certain acupuncture points additionally stimulates the central nervous system, which in turn causes the release of hormones that either affects the perception of pain or generate a sensation of well-being. Get acupuncture therapy administered by a trained and experienced acupuncturist at all times.

Yoga and Stretching

Patients with sciatica frequently report having discomfort after extended sitting or standing, in addition to unexpected and quick moves. The discomfort is further exacerbated by compressing the spine induced by movements such as lifting the legs up, drawing the knees up toward the chest, or squatting. Contrarily, stretching and yoga can assist in stretching your spine and in response, lessen the symptoms of sciatica-induced tightness, inflammation, and back pain.

Garlic

Garlic has anti-inflammatory power, which makes it an effective treatment for sciatica pain. Its anti-inflammation property is quite effective in reducing the pain and inflammation that affect people with sciatica. In addition, to that, the botanicals in garlic can aid in the treatment of low back pain.

Direction

- ✓ 10 garlic cloves, one cup of water, two cups of milk, and some honey should be set aside.

- ✓ In a pan, combine all the ingredients, excluding the honey, and then boil it.

- ✓ Simmer for five minutes and then sieve the content.

- ✓ Allow it to cool slightly and then add the honey.

- ✓ Drink one cup twice daily.

Every element of elderberry, whether it be the fruit, leaves, or flowers, is quite useful. It has the capacity to relax muscles, lowering pressure on the nerve ends. Because it helps to naturally lessen pain and inflammation, it may help to relieve symptoms of sciatica.

Directions

- ✓ Add a teaspoon of elderberry to a cup of hot water and let it steep for fifteen minutes.

- ✓ You may consider adding some honey as a sweetener.

- ✓ strain and consume it three times daily.

Celery

Celery juice is a fantastic method to efficiently treat nerve pain in the body. Because it has anti-inflammatory and antioxidant qualities, it may help to reduce the pain and inflammation related to sciatica.

Directions

- ✓ A few fresh celery leaves should be finely chopped.

- ✓ Add some water to these pieces and blend.

- ✓ Add some honey to improve the juice's flavor before drinking it.

- ✓ It is best to have a cup of celery juice twice daily.

Magnesium is necessary for healthy nerve function. One of the finest ways to quickly access it is by using Epsom salt. This substance is easily absorbed by the skin.

Directions

- ✓ Put hot water in your bathtub.

- ✓ Add 2 cups of Epsom salt after that.

- ✓ Every day for thirty minutes, soak the affected area in this solution to ease symptoms and help the muscles relax.

Horseradish has natural anti-inflammatories and healing effects that can quickly relieve inflammation and ease sciatica pain.

Directions

- ✓ Cut up some horseradish to make a puree

- ✓ Before applying it to your painful area, warm it up slightly.

- ✓ Wrap the area in a clean cloth and let the paste on for two hours.

- ✓ Similarly, you might extract the juice from chopped horseradish.

- ✓ After warming, stir in some honey.

- ✓ Drink two tablespoons of this juice three times each days.

WHEN TO VISIT A DOCTOR

In general, minimal sciatica usually subsides with time. If self-care methods don't ease your discomfort and the pain lasts more than a week, seek medical attention. Ensure you see a doctor immediately you experience any of the following:

- ✓ Both of your legs are affected by sciatica symptoms at the same time.

- ✓ You have paralysis or muscle aches in your leg, thigh, pelvis, or buttocks, as well as deep, acute back or leg discomfort.

- ✓ The discomfort occurs after a serious injury, like a road accident.

- ✓ You are having difficulty managing your bladder and bowel.

- ✓ On your back or around the spine, if you get redness or swelling.

- ✓ You are suffering from back pain and a mysterious fever.

- ✓ You have intense pain that keeps you up at night and gets worse when you lie down.

- ✓ You feel like you're burning when you urinate, or you detect blood in your urine.

- ✓ Intense, paralyzing pain interferes with your usual life and prevents you from executing even the simplest basic tasks notwithstanding good rest, therapy, and workout.

- ✓ Consult your physician if your symptoms don't change after using natural remedies.

✓ If your symptoms worsen over time, you might be dealing with the root of the issue

✓ You feel unexpected acute pain in your lower back or leg.

TIPS TO HELP MANAGE SCIATICA

i.   Avoid making abrupt movements.

ii.   Embrace good postures to alleviate pressure on the lower back.

iii.   Do proper lifting techniques with your knees bent and back straight.

iv.   Sleep on the bed which is not too soft or too firm.

v.   Practice regular exercise and yet avoid engaging in intense exercise.

vi.   Do not smoke cigarettes because it promotes disc degeneration.

vii.   To keep your body balanced and hydrated and to prevent constipation and other medical conditions that could trigger sciatica symptoms, consume enough water on a daily basis.

viii. To aid in your body's quicker recovery, maintain a balanced diet.

ix. The combination of certain fruits, such as pomegranate, lemon, and orange, might enhance the immune system and lessen sciatica nerve inflammation.

x. Incorporate fiber-rich foods into your daily diet to prevent constipation which could endanger your sciatica health more.

CONCLUSION

Sciatica is frequently confused with common back pain. But sciatica is not just a back problem. Being the lengthiest and broadest nerves in the human body, the sciatic nerve runs from the lower back down each leg, ending at the soles of the feet.

Consequently, the piercing pain connected with the constriction or aggravation of the sciatic nerve spreads along the same line, beginning in the lower back and ending at the bases of the big toes of the feet.

Luckily, there is a sciatica pain treatment that may be carried out at home. It's crucial that you see a doctor if any of the at-home solutions don't help your pain decrease. If the pain worsens, you might have a more serious situation than you initially believed.